FAST FACTS

Multiple Sclerosis

Indispensable

Guides to

Clinical

Practice

George D Perkin

Consultant Neurologist, West London
Neurosciences Centre, The Hammersmith
Hospitals NHS Trust, London, UK

Jerry S Wolinsky

Professor of Neurology, The University of
Texas-Houston, Health Science Center,
Houston, Texas, USA

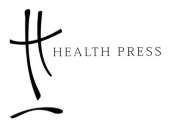

HEALTH PRESS

Oxford

Fast Facts – Multiple Sclerosis
First published 2000

Text © 2000 George D Perkin, Jerry S Wolinsky
© 2000 in this edition Health Press Limited
Health Press Limited, Elizabeth House, Queen Street, Abingdon,
Oxford OX14 3JR, UK

Tel: +44 (0) 1235 523233
Fax: +44 (0) 1235 523238

Fast Facts is a trade mark of Health Press Limited.

The publisher and the authors have made every effort to ensure the
accuracy of this book, but cannot accept responsibility for any errors
or omissions.

A CIP catalogue record for this title is available from the British Library.

ISBN 1-899541-28-4

Perkin, GD (George)
Fast Facts – Multiple Sclerosis/
George D Perkin, Jerry S Wolinsky

Illustrated by MeDee Art, London, UK.

Printed by Fine Print (Services) Ltd, Oxford, UK.

Introduction 5

Epidemiology, pathology and pathophysiology 7

Classification, presentation and early stages 14

The established condition 25

Diagnosis 31

Treatment of acute attacks and symptomatic measures 38

Treatment with immunomodulators 46

Paramedical staff and support groups 53

Future trends 60

Appendix: useful addresses 62

Key references 64

Index 67

Introduction

Until relatively recently, the diagnosis of multiple sclerosis was often subject to error and its treatment, apart from symptomatic measures, largely confined to short-term injections or steroid tablets. With the advent of MRI, more accurate diagnosis became possible. Furthermore, for the first time, it became possible to recognize the very early stages of the disease. More recently, the opportunity to alter the long-term natural history of the disease has been provided by the introduction of the group of interferon drugs and glatiramer acetate.

The publication of *Fast Facts – Multiple Sclerosis* is, therefore, particularly timely. It should prove of considerable value to family physicians, helping them recognize the early stages of multiple sclerosis and reviewing the recent developments in disease management. Nurses and paramedical staff involved in the care of multiple sclerosis patients will also find the book invaluable.

CHAPTER 1
Epidemiology, pathology and pathophysiology

Multiple sclerosis (MS) is a disease characterized by recurrent or chronically progressive neurological dysfunction. It is caused by perivenular inflammatory foci in the white matter of the central nervous system (CNS). Repeated episodes result in characteristic widespread, demyelinated and sclerotic lesions or plaques throughout the brain, optic nerves and spinal cord of affected individuals. An immune-mediated component is central to disease pathogenesis.

Epidemiology

MS is the most common non-traumatic, disabling neurological disease that occurs in young adults. Overall, the prevalence is about 100 cases per 100 000. This amounts to about 350 000 cases in the USA and Canada, and an almost equal number of cases in the UK and Europe. However, the incidence of the disease varies markedly according to age, gender, geography and genetic background. The disease has its peak onset at about 30 years of age, with fewer than 10% of all cases having an onset before puberty or after age 55. Women are disproportionately represented in all series, with a ratio of about 2:1.

The disease shows a geographical gradient of prevalence, with more cases found at the northern latitudes of Europe and North America and at the southern latitudes of New Zealand and Australia. This variation strongly suggests that environmental factors are involved somehow in the pathogenesis of the disease. Migration studies that attribute risk to residence during childhood and the description of apparent disease epidemics support this hypothesis. Caucasians, particularly those of Scandinavian ancestry, have a high risk of the disease, though few ethnic groups are spared.

While increased MS risk is conferred by the DRB1*1501 (DR2) major histocompatibility haplotype, multiple genetic loci are likely to contribute interactively to the risk. The DR molecules are critical in the processing and presentation of foreign and self-antigens to the immune system. Table 1.1 is helpful for counselling family members of newly diagnosed patients.

TABLE 1.1

Age-adjusted risks of familial MS*

Relationship to index case	Male index (%)	Female index (%)
Parents	2.6	3.0
Children	2.5	2.6
Siblings	3.8	4.0
First cousins	1.5	2.4

*Data from Sadovnick *et al.* 1988

Pathology

Plaques are the hallmark pathology of MS, and can occur at any site where there are myelinated axons within the CNS. Myelin is a complex extension of the cytoplasmic membranes of oligodendroglial cells, which cover the large-diameter axons of the CNS. Myelinated axons are able to conduct impulses at rapid rates. High rates are necessary for successful transfer of information between neurones to allow coordinated motor movements, sensory perception and facile cognition. Most often, plaques are found in periventricular locations, within the optic nerves and spinal cord, and in the subcortical white matter of the cerebral hemispheres (Figure 1.1, pages 10 and 11). The distribution of the lesions varies considerably from case to case, mirroring in part the varied clinical presentations of the disease.

Individual plaques show variable amounts of perivenular and parenchymal mononuclear cell inflammation, demyelination with relative axonal sparing, oligodendroglial cell loss and astrocytic proliferation with gliosis (Figure 1.2, pages 12 and 13). It is likely that there are several stages of lesion formation, with plaques characterized as acute, subacute and chronic. Initially, a perivascular infiltrate of T cells and macrophages predominates. The inflamed vascular endothelium expresses a number of molecules that attract additional cells. Also, the endothelium, which normally acts as a barrier to many blood-borne molecules entering the brain, is focally disrupted. In these disrupted areas, the myelin is engulfed by macrophages and actively degraded. Numerous macrophages are found that contain myelin-breakdown products, including myelin proteins and lipids. Some oligodendrocytes persist, and these may attempt to remyelinate neighbouring demyelinated axons. However, most oligodendrocytes within these lesions show cytolytic changes and die. Astrocytes are activated and some demyelinated axons are transected. The axons that are transected are unable to re-establish distant connections, leading to irreversible neurological dysfunction. Chronic lesions show little inflammation, an absence of oligodendroglial cells (except at their extreme margins), and an intense astrogliosis. In some chronic lesions, axonal loss can be marked.

Pathophysiology

Electrical conduction and signal transmission along the larger axons of the CNS is facilitated by the formation of internodes, which have a high concentration of sodium channels, along the axon. The internodal regions are separated by heavily myelinated segments. During MS attacks, active demyelination results in a failure of impulse transmission across the demyelinated axon segments, causing the associated symptoms. Conduction is restored by remyelination, which re-establishes a near-normal internodal architecture; the clinical attack subsequently regresses. However, the factors that contribute to conduction block and the restoration of effective, if not normal, conduction are more complicated than this simple construct. Neuro-electrical blocking factors in serum, re-organization of sodium channels along demyelinated nodes, and other factors are also likely to account for the loss and return of clinical function in the face of chronic demyelination. Conversely, axonal loss is highly correlated with non-reversible neurological impairment.

Some of the events that contribute to lesion formation are now reasonably well understood. During the course of any viral infection, macrophages take up the viral proteins and degrade them into their individual antigenic components. The component fragments are recognized by the immune system. The antigens are presented as protein fragments on the surfaces of macrophages by their DR molecules. Normally, the presentation of these antigens to the immune system leads to the activation of T cells, which begins a cascade that results in elimination of the virus. However, in MS, it is postulated that a portion of the responding cells mistakes the viral antigen for a self-protein, probably a protein found in

(a)

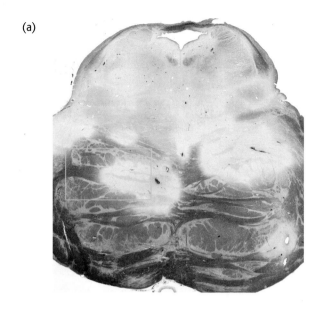

Figure 1.1 Different staining techniques used to demonstrate plaques in the brain of a patient with MS. (a) A section through the pons at the level of the third nerve nuclei stained specifically for myelin (black). Multiple ovoid areas fail to stain, reflecting the presence of well-developed MS plaques. The region within the yellow box is shown in detail and arrows highlight the same region of crossing fibres in the pons. (b) Stained with haematoxylin and eosin, the crossing fibres are pale as they enter the edge of the plaque. (c) Stained for myelin, there is a loss of staining for the same fibres entering the plaque. (d) Using an axonal silver stain, it is difficult to determine where the plaque is located because of the relative sparing of axons.

myelin. The number of systemically activated effector T cells, the pro-inflammatory CD4+ Th1 cells, increases in the circulation. These then enter the brain at sites with an increased display of surface adhesion molecules on the vascular endothelium to cause further disruption of the blood–brain barrier. Adhesion molecules occur normally on the endothelium, but increase when the endothelium is damaged, attracting T cells and helping them enter the brain. As these cells migrate into the brain and encounter myelin antigens, they secrete a number of cytokines (IL-2, TNFα and IFNγ) and chemokines. These substances recruit antigen-non-specific mononuclear cells, thus amplifying the cascade of myelin-destructive substances in the

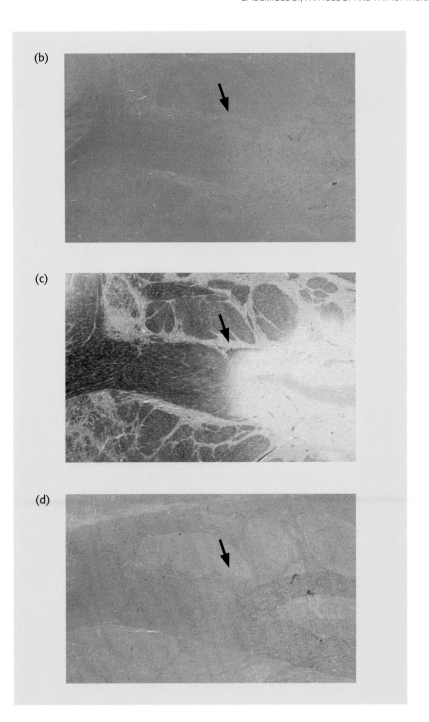

(a)

Large white
matter lesion

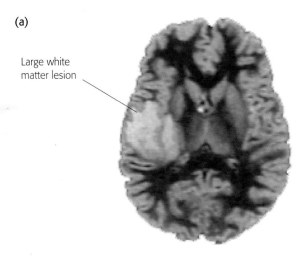

Figure 1.2 A 32-year-old woman presented with several weeks of progressive left-sided numbness. (a) Dual-inversion recovery MRI disclosed a large lesion, restricted to the white matter of the right temporal-parietal region; normal white matter and cerebrospinal fluid (CSF) appear dark, and grey matter structures appear light grey. A cerebral biopsy was performed to obtain a definitive diagnosis and eliminate the possibility of a tumour. (b) (Facing page) Tissue staining with haematoxylin and eosin disclosed a sea of macrophages separated by strands of the cytoplasm of reactive astrocytes (arrowed). (c) Staining with Luxol fast blue showed that macrophage cytoplasm contained recently degraded myelin, stained purple (arrowed). Staining for axons showed their relative preservation in the biopsy material (not shown). A few small high-signal-intensity lesions were found in the white matter of the opposite hemisphere and examination of CSF disclosed 47 lymphocytes, an increased immunoglobulin G synthetic rate and a single oligoclonal band. Her symptoms resolved following treatment with intravenous methylprednisolone and she responded well to interferon therapy. Massive demyelinating lesions of this type are uncommon and, when solitary, mimic tumours and may have a monophasic disease course.

region of the developing lesion. This intense, perivenular inflammation is associated with local disruption of the blood–brain barrier, the development of vasogenic oedema, and the influx of myelinotoxic substances from the blood, including certain immunoglobulins and complement factors. Macrophages and activated microglia engulf and degrade myelin, stripping it from axons that traverse the lesion. With intense activity, oligodendroglia are lost and axons are transected. However, in some lesions, despite active myelin breakdown, surviving oligodendroglia can remyelinate those demyelinated axons that survive.

It is likely that another type of T cell, CD4+ Th2, which secretes regulatory cytokines (IL-4 and TGFβ), eventually suppresses the inflammatory response and limits damage. Major changes in regional vascular permeability resolve over weeks, and myelin-breakdown products are removed over months. As the inflammation subsides, only scant inflammatory cells remain. These are often immunoglobulin-secreting B cells. Astrocytes are activated early in lesion formation, and contribute to the intense gliosis, which is the type of scarring that occurs in the CNS and characterizes many chronic plaques. The destructive process is repeated in an unpredictable manner in previously unaffected regions of CNS white matter. It can also recur at sites of remyelination or incomplete demyelination, and can extend at the edges of chronic lesions, involving more white matter over time.

Activation of systemic, pro-inflammatory CD4+ Th1 cells can follow a variety of non-specific viral infections. These infections are the well-recognized precipitants of clinical attacks. However, the events that initiate the unregulated expansion of putative antigen-specific T cells, or trigger the influx of these cells into the brain, are unknown. Similarly, it is unclear if the immunoregulatory abnormalities that have been demonstrated repeatedly in patients with MS are primary or secondary to an abnormality in CNS-myelin maintenance, as might be seen with a persistent viral infection.

(b)   (c)

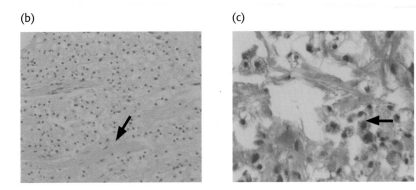

Figure 1.2 Continued.

CHAPTER 2
Classification, presentation and early stages

The major types of MS, based on distinctive clinical presentations, are:
- remitting relapsing disease
- secondary progressive disease
- primary progressive disease
- progressive relapsing disease.

Of these, remitting relapsing and secondary progressive are by far the most common types. Primary progressive disease occurs in no more than 15% of all MS patients, and fewer than 5% of MS patients have the progressive relapsing form. While these disease subtypes can be easily described, many patients fit poorly into these major disease categories. Furthermore, there is little evidence to suggest that important differences exist in the underlying pathophysiology of any of these four disease types. The best distinction is between the relapsing forms of the disease (i.e. remitting relapsing and secondary progressive) and primary progressive disease, where certain MRI characteristics often differ. Whether these currently accepted standard definitions will withstand scrutiny or lead to a better understanding of MS as a disease process is presently unsettled.

Prodromal symptoms
It has been suggested that, in many cases, the initial neurological presentation of MS is preceded by non-specific complaints, such as fatigue, altered appetite, mood change or memory disturbance. As most patients attending out-patient departments tend to have such symptoms, their specificity is open to question!

Remitting relapsing disease
This is, by far, the most common form of MS at presentation. Characteristically, patients experience acute attacks of neurological dysfunction. However, it is rare for the neurological symptoms and signs to develop in an apoplectic fashion. More commonly, symptoms of neurological dysfunction increase over a number of days to several weeks, reaching a maximum deficit which, if untreated, persists for several days to

several weeks before complete or incomplete recovery occurs over a matter of weeks to months. Recovery from these discrete attacks or relapses is typically most rapid and most complete at disease onset. Several definitions of the acute attack have been suggested, particularly for uniformity in clinical trial design and conduct. These also serve the clinician well.

Definition. The following define a clinical attack.

- New or recurrent neurological signs and symptoms, which last at least 48 hours.
- These symptoms must occur following an interval of at least 30 days of stable neurological function.
- As MS patients may experience transient recurrence of symptoms from prior attacks during any metabolic insult or with a fever, the new or recurrent symptoms and signs must appear in the absence of fever, intercurrent infection or other significant metabolic derangements.
- Finally, most clinical trials require demonstration of objective signs of neurological dysfunction reasonably referable to involvement of central myelinated pathways.

In general, clinicians are well advised to follow this last rule. This requirement is most readily fulfilled by objective examination of the patient when his or her symptoms suggest motor, visual or coordination pathway involvement. It can often be difficult to substantiate when the patient's symptoms are solely sensory. Often, well-reported symptoms of numbness in an arm or leg lack objective confirmation on neurological examination, even though they may reflect significant attacks to the patient.

The definition of remitting relapsing disease type does not require the return of normal, symptom-free neurological function following an attack. However, any residual symptoms, neurological findings or disability acquired during an attack must remain stable between attacks. In this form of the disease, any accumulation of neurological deterioration must occur in a stepwise fashion, in the wake of well-defined acute exacerbations or relapses. These two patterns of remitting relapsing disease, relapses with return to normal neurological function and relapsing disease with stepwise, accumulated disability are shown in Figure 2.1. The distribution of initial symptoms in one early series is given in Table 2.1. Acute presenting symptoms typical of remitting relapsing MS take many forms.

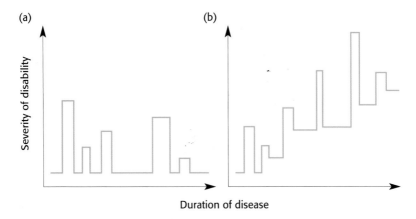

Figure 2.1 The two patterns of remitting relapsing disease: (a) relapses with return to normal neurological function; (b) relapsing disease with stepwise, accumulated disability.

TABLE 2.1

Initial symptoms in an early series of patients with remitting relapsing MS

Initial symptom	Incidence (%)
Weakness	40
Loss of vision	22
Paraesthesiae	21
Diplopia	12
Vertigo	5
Altered micturition	5

Presenting symptoms

Weakness. Acute weakness of the lower limbs is the presenting complaint in some patients. However, many of these patients with myelitis and, in effect, complete cord transection seldom show evidence of MS during a protracted follow-up period. An episode of heaviness in one or both lower limbs, or a complaint of exercise-induced weakness and heaviness of the lower limbs are more common presenting features (Case history 2.1). Examination may show little in such cases save, perhaps, depression of the abdominal reflexes, or an extensor plantar response on one side.

Case history 2.1

A 45-year-old woman developed a loss of reactivity in her right leg 4 months prior to presentation. The leg failed to respond properly when she tried to move it. It felt heavy and she began to trip. She noticed slight weakness and clumsiness of the right hand with a loss of precision in her writing. On examination, the reflexes were slightly brisker in the right arm than the left and there was slight loss of right-hand dexterity. There was some weakness in the right leg and the reflexes were slightly brisker in the right leg compared with the left. The plantars were flexor. MRI and her subsequent history established a diagnosis of MS.

Loss of vision typically occurs as part of an attack of acute optic neuritis. In most patients, pain appears in or around the eye, and is usually exacerbated by eye movement. Shortly afterwards, visual loss occurs. The degree of loss of vision varies – some patients effectively become blind in the affected eye. Findings include a field defect (predominantly central in most) and an abnormal pupillary light response (Figure 2.2). The optic disc may be swollen and is sometimes surrounded by haemorrhages. Visual recovery occurs in the majority, over a median period of about 8 weeks.

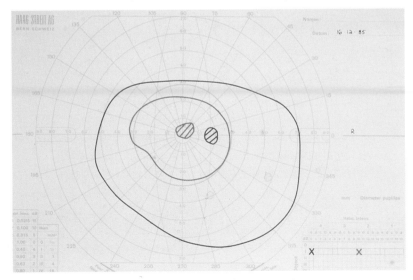

Figure 2.2 Right central scotoma in a patient with optic neuritis.

Paraesthesiae occur in characteristic patterns that may spread from one leg to the other and then to a level on the trunk, or altered sensation in the periphery of one or more limbs (Case history 2.2). Objective findings may be slight, but enquiry about symptoms induced by neck flexion is worthwhile. Some patients, even as a presenting feature, will complain that neck flexion leads to a shower of paraesthesiae ('electric shocks') radiating down the spine into the legs (Lhermitte's phenomenon). Though the symptom (which is associated with pathology in the cervical spinal cord) occurs in several conditions, its presence in a young person almost always indicates MS if cervical trauma has been excluded.

Diplopia may occur as an isolated symptom at the onset of MS, or be part of a more global disturbance of brainstem function (Figure 2.3). Sometimes an abducens palsy is responsible. Isolated palsies of the third cranial nerve are uncommon in MS, and those of the fourth cranial nerve are virtually unknown. Some patients with diplopia will have evidence of an internuclear ophthalmoplegia, though more commonly they describe an ill-defined blurring of vision or a problem with visual tracking. If such patients are asked to re-fix their gaze between two objects in the horizontal plane, the adducting eye is seen to lag behind the abducting eye. The latter eye usually shows a few beats of nystagmus. The problem may affect gaze to one or both sides. The physical sign, in young people, is almost pathognomonic of MS.

Case history 2.2

A 23-year-old woman awoke 12 days before consultation with itching sensations in both hands, followed by an awareness of loss of temperature sensitivity in the right hand only. Later, this spread to the right shoulder, trunk and parts of the right leg. Examination revealed loss of pain and temperature sensation on the right side with a level at about C5. The sacral dermatomes were spared. Her cerebrospinal fluid examination was normal, and she recovered.

Four years later, the patient developed altered sensation in the legs and right side of her face. On examination, the findings were compatible with a fresh disturbance of the sensory pathways.

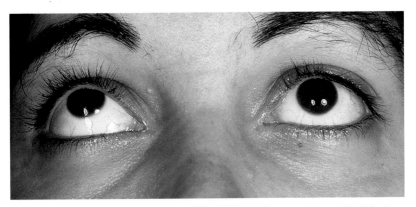

Figure 2.3 Impaired vertical gaze in the left eye in a patient presenting with diplopia.

Vertigo. In young people, vertigo is far more likely to be associated with a disorder of the vestibular apparatus in the inner ear than its central connections. If vertigo is triggered by head movement, the accompanying nystagmus tends not to fatigue, and to be triggered by movements in different directions, thereby distinguishing it from benign positional vertigo. In most patients, there are likely to be additional symptoms, such as diplopia or facial numbness, that signal the origin of the symptom.

Altered micturition. Though the majority of MS patients have altered micturition by the time the disease is fully developed, it is unusual for disturbed sphincter control to be an early feature. Symptoms include hesitancy or urgency or a mixture, explicable on the basis of a mismatch between bladder wall contraction and failure of relaxation of the bladder neck (Case history 2.3). Disturbance of bowel control in the early stages is rare.

Symptoms triggered by certain activities. One-third of patients with fully developed MS will describe a transient exacerbation of their symptoms triggered by certain activities, particularly walking and hot baths (Uhthoff's phenomenon; Case history 2.4). The basis of this probably lies in blockage of conduction in partly demyelinated nerve fibres in the relevant fibre pathway when body temperature rises. In some instances, exercise-induced symptoms are the first manifestation of the disease; symptoms appear during exercise and are then rapidly relieved by rest. Patients with this particular presentation tend to have a primary progressive rather than remitting relapsing form of the disease.

Case history 2.3

A 33-year-old woman had a 2-week history of ill-defined back pain and slight numbness in her legs. For 2 days, she had had difficulty with micturition, leading to retention for which she was catheterized. Bowel function, and vaginal, urethral and buttock sensation were normal. Examination showed depressed abdominal responses, just-detectable lower limb spasticity and bilateral extensor plantar responses. MRI showed signal changes compatible with MS. The patient received a course of corticosteroids and recovered.

Case history 2.4

For a year, this 27-year-old man had noticed visual blurring when walking, the left eye being more affected than the right. His eyesight recovered after resting for about 30 minutes. The same problem, accompanied by weakness and unsteadiness of the legs, occurred when he took a hot bath. On examination, there was left optic disc pallor and bilateral lower limb spasticity with extensor plantar responses. Investigations established a diagnosis of MS.

Paroxysmal symptoms have been described in MS patients (Table 2.2). These may appear during the course of the disease or at the outset. The features of trigeminal neuralgia in MS do not distinguish it from the type of neuralgia occurring in older subjects, except that bilateral symptoms are more likely in MS. While it is usually considered that the neuralgia is triggered by MS lesions in the pons close to the entry zone of the trigeminal nerve, some cases, as is usual with older subjects, appear to be due to cross-compression by blood vessels in the posterior fossa.

All the paroxysmal symptoms are characterized by their frequency (up to 100 attacks per day, for example), their stereotyped nature, their brevity (seconds usually) and their response to carbamazepine. After a period of days or weeks, but seldom longer, the episodes remit.

Rarer presentations. The following are less common presenting symptoms.

TABLE 2.2

Paroxysmal symptoms

- Trigeminal neuralgia
- Dysarthria and ataxia
- Tonic seizures
- Paraesthesiae
- Pain
- Itching

- Altered intellectual function is well recognized in MS, particularly in its later stages. A sub-cortical dementia has been described, characterized by a slowing of information processing but with little or no evidence of cortical features, such as aphasia, apraxia or agnosia. Rarely, dementia may be prominent at the outset.
- Mood disturbance is common, and is far more likely to manifest as depression than euphoria. There is no firm evidence that such problems are the initial feature of the disease.
- Epilepsy occurs more commonly in MS patients than in controls. It seldom appears at the outset.
- A presentation mimicking a brain tumour is recognized. Features include a rapidly evolving hemiparesis or dysphasia, accompanied by headache. CT or MRI, particularly the former, may increase the confusion by showing a ring-enhancing lesion (Figure 2.4).

Progression. About 30% of all patients with MS will still be classified as having remitting relapsing disease at 25 years after initial diagnosis of the condition. About two-thirds of patients who remain remitting relapsing in type will have limited accumulated neurological findings and little actual disability from their disease. This subset of patients can be considered to have benign disease, a form of MS that cannot be prospectively defined.

Secondary progressive disease
This form of MS invariably evolves from the remitting relapsing disease type. While most patients initially present with remitting relapsing disease,

21

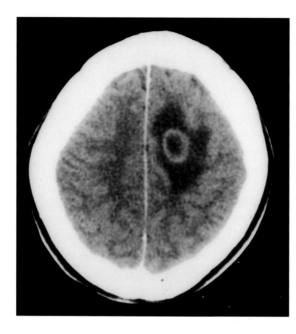

Figure 2.4
A CT scan showing a ring-enhancing lesion in a patient with MS.

a substantial proportion eventually develop secondary progressive disease. Here, neurological disability accumulates over time, with or without continued superimposed acute relapses.

Definition. The following aspects are critical to the definition of this disease type.

- The patient must have had prior well-documented or well-recalled episodes of acute attacks of MS before entering a phase of accumulated disability.
- Symptoms, neurological signs and disability from the disease accumulate in gradual or accelerated fashion in the absence of attacks, or between well-delineated relapses.
- Patients who enter the secondary progressive phase of disease may or may not continue to have relapses. These two subcategories of secondary progressive disease are illustrated in Figure 2.5.

Progression. Large clinical series of untreated MS patients suggest that about half of all patients will develop the secondary progressive form of the disease within 7–9 years of diagnosis. Nearly 70% of all patients with MS eventually enter a progressive phase of their illness.

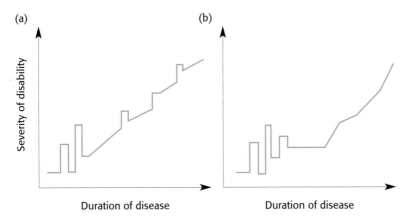

Figure 2.5 In secondary progressive MS, patients (a) may or (b) may not continue to have relapses.

Primary progressive disease

This is characterized by slowly accumulated neurological disability without prior or current well-defined attacks of neurological dysfunction. Patients with this form of disease often present with symptoms suggesting progressive spinal cord dysfunction with lower limb weakness, tightness and reduced gait endurance. They commonly have urinary frequency and urgency. Whereas females predominate with relapsing presentations, males and older women are more likely to present with progressive disease from the onset. Because of the prominent symptoms suggesting spinal cord dysfunction, a careful search for conditions that cause progressive myelopathy is required (Case history 2.5).

Case history 2.5

A 60-year-old man had a progressive problem with walking, over 18 months. He described a loss of flexibility of the left leg, finding lifting it particularly difficult. He was unable to run. His hands became clumsier. Examination showed dysarthria, poor lateral tongue movements and a spastic tetraparesis. There was mild upper and lower limb ataxia, and vibration sense in the feet was absent. Further investigation established a diagnosis of MS.

Characteristically, patients with progressive disease have difficulty determining if they are worsening on a day-to-day, week-to-week or even a month-to-month basis. They are usually able to determine worsening in relation to major milestones, such as from one year's holiday to the next. The type of things a patient is no longer able to accomplish becomes evident. The tempo of disease progression is usually slow and ingravescent, but may be punctuated by intervals in which the patient appears quite stable, experiences some improvement for no clear reason, or shows a more accelerated deterioration of function overall.

Sometimes, when careful histories of patients with the progressive presentation are taken, they may recall an isolated episode of neurological dysfunction, such as optic neuritis, that may have preceded the development of progressive neurological disability by one or more decades. Often, these patients have not sought medical attention for the remote symptoms, or a definite diagnosis has never been reached. By strict definition, such individuals have secondary progressive MS.

Progressive relapsing disease

This uncommon disease type is characterized by an initial course that simulates primary progression, but with one or more clearly defined, superimposed attack that appears after the progressive disease is well established. Typical patterns of primary progressive and progressive relapsing disease are illustrated in Figure 2.6.

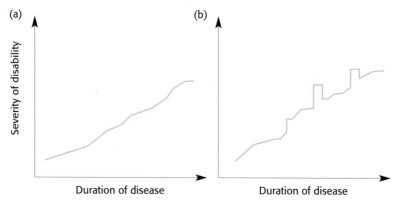

Figure 2.6 Typical patterns of disease in (a) primary progressive and (b) progressive relapsing MS.

CHAPTER 3

The established condition

The features of established MS depend, to some extent, on the way in which the condition originally presented as well as its mode of progression. A useful visual format displays the patient's disability against time (Figure 3.1). For patients with benign MS, the established condition is, in a sense, not established at all, since those patients, even 15 or 20 years after presentation, have little or no disability, little or no restriction of activity, and indeed seldom present themselves for medical attention, at least in the UK.

As has been discussed in Chapter 2, although the majority of patients with MS present with a remitting and relapsing picture, many of these patients

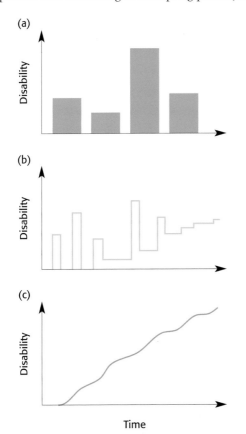

Figure 3.1

Relationship of disability severity to duration of disease in (a) benign remitting relapsing MS, (b) remitting relapsing MS with secondary progression, and (c) primary progressive MS.

enter a secondary progressive phase, in which relapse frequency lessens, but residual disability emerges between attacks, and then slowly progresses.

Most studies agree that relapse frequency is highest in the first few years of the disease. There is little evidence that relapse frequency influences outcome, but considerable data indicate that the interval between the initial attack and the first relapse is significant. As this period lengthens, the likelihood of benign MS increases.

Eventually, whether in primary progressive or secondary progressive MS, a fairly consistent pattern emerges, with an attendant level of disability (Figure 3.2). Figures for the rate of progression of the disease and its effect on lifespan vary considerably, however.

Mental function

Altered mental function is commonplace in the established condition. Indeed, studies now suggest that subtle changes of intellectual function may appear quite early. In some patients, a picture of progressive intellectual

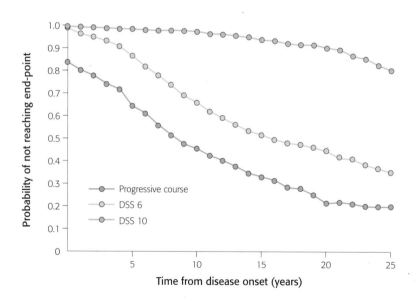

Figure 3.2 The rate at which certain end-points are reached during the course of MS. DSS 6 = walking 100 metres with assistance, e.g. with a cane or walker; DSS 10 = death related to the MS process. Adapted from Runmarker and Andersen 1993.

impairment, aligned with a gait disorder mimics the presentation of normal pressure hydrocephalus (Case history 3.1). Depression is far more common than euphoria in the established condition.

Visual function

After some years of the disease, many patients will have pallor of part or the whole of one or both optic discs, regardless of whether they have had attacks of optic neuritis (Case history 3.2). Despite this, visual acuity is usually preserved.

Case history 3.1

A 46-year-old woman had a 4-year history of progressive cognitive impairment associated with a gait disorder with apraxic features. At times, the disability fluctuated. On examination, her mini-mental test score was 18 out of 30. She had first-degree jerk nystagmus to the right, limb ataxia and extensor plantar responses. Her gait was apraxic, with a tendency to be rooted to the spot, unable to progress either forwards or backwards. Her CSF and MRI findings were typical of MS.

Case history 3.2

This man had been diagnosed as having MS 14 years previously. He had no specific visual complaints. His arms felt strong, but he was aware of tingling and numbness in the fingertips. He was just able to stand with a frame but found walking extremely difficult. His legs were liable to stiffen or jerk. He complained of urgency of micturition coupled with incontinence but, at other times, hesitancy. He had been chronically constipated. He had had erectile impotence for some time. Examination showed optic disc pallor but no other cranial nerve abnormality. His upper limbs were spastic and showed a mild pyramidal weakness coupled with cerebellar ataxia. He had impaired proprioception in the fingers. There was a severe spastic paraparesis with marked impairment of vibration sense throughout the legs and reduced joint position sense in the feet.

Eye movements

An internuclear ophthalmoplegia is the most common persisting oculomotor sign (other than nystagmus) in established MS. The abnormality may be unilateral or bilateral. Patients seldom complain of diplopia, but some will have noticed problems with the tracking of moving objects (Figure 3.3).

Motor function

A small proportion of patients with long-standing MS may show either depressed reflexes or wasting. For most, however, the motor deficit is pyramidal in type and characterized by a spastic paraparesis of varying degree. Typical findings include spastic legs, ankle clonus and bilateral extensor plantar responses. With the passage of time, patients become increasingly reliant either on walking aids or the use of a wheelchair. Upper limb involvement is more variable and, fortunately, seldom reaches a degree that renders the patient totally dependent.

Cerebellar function

Limb ataxia is commonplace in established MS. When it is severe, it interferes substantially with everyday function. Truncal ataxia may be disproportionate to limb involvement, so that the predominant disturbance is of gait. A cerebellar dysarthria is likely if the limb findings are prominent. In addition to nystagmus, cerebellar eye signs include broken pursuit movement and over-shooting or under-shooting saccades. Only rarely is the disability purely cerebellar in the later stages of the disease.

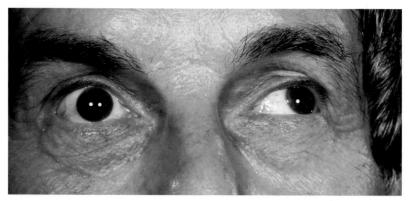

Figure 3.3 Internuclear ophthalmoplegia.

Sphincter function

Bladder symptoms are common in the established condition. Retention is unusual – most patients complain of a mixture of frequency and urgency, often coupled with hesitancy. This curious combination arises out of a mismatch between contraction of the detrusor muscle (triggering the urgency) and failure of sphincter relaxation (triggering the hesitancy). Faecal urgency and incontinence are mercifully uncommon.

Sexual function

Erectile impotence has been found in up to 40% of male patients and correlates with the presence of sphincter impairment.

Questions that patients often ask

Is the disease hereditary? Genetic factors play a part in determining susceptibility to MS (see Table 1.1).

What is the effect of pregnancy? There is no evidence for an increase in relapse frequency during pregnancy itself, but relapse frequency does increase in the first 3 months of the puerperium. There is no evidence of an adverse effect of MS on the fetus, or that long-term outcome of MS is influenced by previous obstetric history.

Can I have vaccinations? There is no firm evidence that single-vaccination procedures trigger an acute exacerbation of MS or alter its long-term outcome.

Can trauma bring on new symptoms? This remains a controversial issue and receives regular airing in courts of law. Despite the fact that some patients describe the development of focal neurological deficit related to the site of recent trauma (Case history 3.3), epidemiological data do not support a link between trauma and the precipitation or worsening of MS.

Can I have an anaesthetic? There is no evidence that anaesthesia, whether general or local, triggers exacerbations of the disease.

Should I go on a diet? There is very little evidence to support dietary change in MS. Many patients move to a diet low in animal fats, with supplements of

29

Case history 3.3

A 19-year-old woman received blows to the left shoulder and face while playing hockey. A few hours later, she developed blurring of vision in the left eye, associated with pain on eye movement. She had had an episode of right optic neuritis 2 years previously. On examination, the right disc was pale, but the left slightly swollen. There was a left relative afferent pupillary defect and visual acuity was reduced to the perception of hand movements only. Vision failed to recover.

---

polyunsaturated fatty acids (e.g. linoleic acid, linolenic acid and arachidonic acid). Favoured supplements include sunflower seed and evening primrose oils. The diets are, in a sense, healthy ones, but there are very little data supporting their use. There is no evidence to support a switch to a gluten-free diet.

Should I have oxygen therapy? Although an early study suggested that hyperbaric (high-pressure) oxygen therapy was beneficial, the findings could not be reproduced.

Can I drive? Regulations vary from country to country. In both the UK and USA, drivers may retain their licence (which normally expires when the driver reaches the age of 70) providing medical assessment has confirmed that driving performance is not impaired. Under certain circumstances, specially adapted vehicles may be recommended. If the diagnosis is recent, or there is evidence of rapid progression, a short-period licence (1, 2 or 3 years) will be issued in the UK. For heavy goods vehicles, a 1-year licence may be issued subject to the condition being stable and there being no driving impairment.

As it is not always possible to judge the influence of neurological disabilities on the ability to respond appropriately in real driving situations, simulated and actual observation under road conditions is often advisable before assuming that one may or may not be able to handle a vehicle securely.

CHAPTER 4
Diagnosis

Diagnosis of MS continues to rest on clinical signs and symptoms. However, paraclinical investigation with modern neuro-imaging and the selected use of electrophysiological testing, together with a careful laboratory analysis of CSF, greatly enhance confidence in the diagnosis. Further, the MRI and CSF findings have a predictive value at first presentation when the clinical diagnosis is suspect.

Clinical criteria

Several different clinical criteria have been proposed. The most widely used are those of the Washington Panel (Table 4.1). While proposed as criteria for use in research trials, they generally serve clinicians well in everyday practice. These criteria are specific for relapsing forms of MS and are not applicable to primary progressive MS where the Schumacher criteria are more relevant.

As applied to patients with primary progressive MS, the Schumacher criteria require:

- sustained progression of neurological disease reasonably referable to disease in CNS white-matter pathways
- onset of symptoms before 55 years of age
- exclusion of competing conditions by appropriate diagnostic studies, including neuro-imaging.

The presence of oligoclonal bands in the CSF is strongly supportive of diagnosis in primary progressive cases. Clearly, great attention to differential diagnosis is required for these individuals.

A revision of the Washington Panel criteria is now required to incorporate advances in MR imaging of MS and to provide integrated criteria for the diagnosis of all clinical forms of MS with similar levels of certainty.

Paraclinical criteria

Neurophysiological tests. Slowing of impulse transmission along rapidly conducting, myelinated, large-fibre pathways is a hallmark of demyelination. Conduction velocities over several CNS sensory pathways can be reproducibly measured using generally available techniques. The selected use

TABLE 4.1

Diagnostic criteria for MS (Washington Panel criteria)

	Relapses*	Clinical lesions**	Separate paraclinical lesions[†]	Oligoclonal bands
Clinically definite	≥ 2	≥ 2	–	–
	2	≥ 1	≥ 1	–
Clinically probable	2	≥ 1	–	–
	1	≥ 2	–	–
	1	≥ 1	≥ 1	–
Laboratory-supported definite	≥ 2	≥ 1	–	≥ 2
	1	≥ 2	–	≥ 2
	1	≥ 1	≥ 1	≥ 2

*Well-documented clinical attacks of dysfunction within CNS white-matter pathways (see Chapter 3)
**Lesions inferred by objective evidence of abnormalities found on examination at the time of diagnosis
[†]Lesions documented by abnormal evoked responses or on MRI distinct from clinical lesions
– = Not required for additional diagnostic certainty at this level

of evoked potentials (visual, auditory and somatosensory) can confirm the diagnosis of MS. However, testing should not duplicate established clinical findings. For example, in a patient with optic neuritis, slowing of conduction on visual-evoked responses does not implicate an additional CNS lesion. In contrast, with a normal neurological examination outside of the visual system, abnormalities on somatosensory-evoked responses provide paraclinical evidence of subclinical involvement of the spinal cord that increases diagnostic certainty (Table 4.1). Magnetic stimulation of the motor cortex can be used to evaluate the integrity of conduction over central pyramidal pathways. Unfortunately, this potentially useful test is not broadly available.

Magnetic resonance imaging is the most useful investigative tool when MS is suspected. It has also greatly advanced our understanding of the dynamics of lesion formation in the disease. Disease activity in relapsing forms of MS, as monitored by serial MRI, is five to ten times more frequent than is suggested by clinical attack rates. As a neuro-imaging modality, MRI has great sensitivity for detecting the types of lesions seen in MS. Unfortunately, the abnormalities found on MRI – particularly those seen on a single examination – are not specific for the disease. Nonetheless, while not often present early in the clinical course, certain combinations of findings on cerebral MRI have high specificity for MS (Table 4.2). Selective imaging of the spinal cord and optic nerves may be useful in some patients. However, as with neurophysiological testing, directed examination of these areas is more fruitful in individual cases, for example, when anatomical definition of lesions is required for differential diagnostic purposes. In general, cerebral MRI alone is most cost-effective for routine initial diagnosis.

Lesions are most often represented by high-signal-intensity ovoids in periventricular and subcortical white matter on T2-weighted images. Active lesions show enhancement on T1-weighted images following the administration of paramagnetic contrast agents composed of irreversible chelates of gadolinium. Some lesions are seen as regions of reduced signal intensity on T1-weighted images. When these lesions persist over multiple examinations, they signify chronic plaques that pathologically show substantial tissue disruption and axonal loss. These persistent

TABLE 4.2

Possible criteria for clinically definite MS by magnetic resonance imaging

T2-weighted sequences	≥ 3 high-signal-intensity lesions in cerebral white matter
	≥ 1 lesion of ≥ 5 mm in isolated cerebral white matter
	≥ 1 lesion in white matter of posterior fossa structures
	≥ 1 ovoid-shaped lesion adjacent to and perpendicular to the lateral ventricle
	≥ 1 subcortical U-fibre lesion
T1-weighted post-gadolinium sequences	≥ 1 enhanced lesion, but not all the lesions seen on T2-weighted images at same session
	≥ 1 unenhanced low-signal-intensity lesion

The diagnostic sensitivity of MRI falls as the number of criteria increases, but the specificity of the diagnosis rises as more criteria are fulfilled 'dark holes' correlate with greater clinical disability. Typical lesions in clinically definite MS found by MRI are shown in Figure 4.1.

Laboratory criteria

A number of immunological and immunochemical abnormalities occur in MS patients as a group, but none discriminates individual patients from those with other neurological diseases or from healthy individuals. All CSF

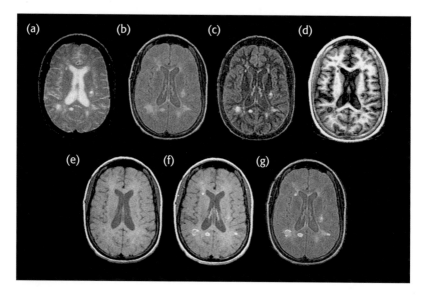

Figure 4.1 MR images from a 39-year-old woman with remitting relapsing MS and an extended disability status score of 1.5. She had experienced increased fatigue and new numbness and clumsiness of her right leg. MS was suspected when she experienced her first bout of sensory symptoms and mild sensory loss 11 years earlier. The MRI slices shown were taken using the following pulse sequences: (a) T2-weighted; (b) FLAIR (fluid attenuation by inversion recovery); (c) dual-inversion recovery for the suppression of normal white matter and CSF; (d) dual-inversion recovery for the suppression of grey matter and CSF; (e) unenhanced T1-weighted; (f) post-gadolinium-enhanced T1-weighted; (g) a composite image of the map of the gadolinium-enhanced tissue (yellow) superimposed onto the FLAIR images of the lesions. Some of the MS plaques are enhanced, signifying inflammatory activity. Many have different appearances on images obtained by different sequences, regardless of their enhancement status. This variable pattern is characteristic of MS.

abnormalities are non-specific. However, in an appropriate clinical setting, some CSF parameters are very useful for increasing the likelihood of diagnosis.

In MS, the CSF often shows a mild, mononuclear-cell pleocytosis and total protein is slightly elevated. However, more than 50 cells per mm^3 or protein content above 100 mg per 100 ml are unusual findings in MS and should alert suspicion of an alternative diagnosis. Myelin basic protein (MBP) and other myelin proteins are released into the CSF during several processes that damage myelin, and can be measured. Intrathecal synthesis of immunoglobulin is always an abnormal finding. This is measurable with increasing sensitivity by determination of:

- CSF gamma globulins as a percentage of total protein
- an index of the amount of CSF immunoglobulin G normalized to the amount of CSF and serum albumin and immunoglobulin G
- CSF immunoglobulin G synthetic rate.

The immunoglobulin G index and synthetic rates are highly reproducible in commercial laboratories. However, finding bands of limited heterogeneity (i.e. oligoclonal bands) is very technique dependent, and sensitivity varies with the experience and care of the reference laboratory. In research centres, oligoclonal bands are found in approximately 95% of patients with clinically definite MS. At diagnosis, CSF evaluation is most helpful in those patients with clinically probable MS (Table 4.1), or who are suspected of having primary progressive disease.

Clinical staging

While not routinely used in clinical practice, a number of scales have been adopted to attempt to stage the accumulation of neurological findings, disability and impairment in patients with MS. These have primarily been developed for use in clinical trials. All the scales have a number of significant limitations. Nevertheless, the expanded disability status score (EDSS) has been used so often that it has attained, by default, gold-standard status for the judgement of clinical trial outcomes. In order to understand the results of current clinical trials and to put individual patients into perspective regarding natural history studies, it is useful to have some working knowledge of the EDSS system, even if it is not universally embraced in the day-to-day management of patients.

Expanded disability status score. The EDSS is gained from the neurological examination supplemented by a formalized assessment of symptoms, and an evaluation of the patient's global abilities, such as to walk or transfer independently, or with help. Recent clinical studies have put additional restrictions and definitions on the original EDSS that are designed to improve its reproducibility when applied by different investigators in multicentre trials. Some of these changes are subtle and others more obvious, but all may lead to somewhat different behaviour of the scoring system, which may account for variations in outcome between studies using similar therapeutic agents.

The classic EDSS is an amalgamation of scoring in eight predefined functional systems:

- pyramidal
- sensory
- cerebellar
- bowel and bladder
- brainstem
- visual
- mental.

A last category of 'other' functions is also included, but is poorly defined. Scoring of the functional systems ranges from normal (0) to severe disabilities (5 or 6 depending on the system). The EDSS ranges from 0 (a patient with a normal neurological examination and no bowel or bladder symptoms) to 10 (a patient who has died due to their MS), with 18 intermediate steps at 0.5 unit increments from 1.0.

- EDSS levels from 0 to 1.5 reflect neurological findings without associated disability.
- Levels from 2.0 to 3.0 include neurological findings with the patient aware of some mild disability.
- Levels 3.5 and 4.0 reflect increasing disability in one or more functional system, but with generally an unrestricted gait and good endurance.
- Levels 5.0 and 5.5 reflect the distance that one can walk without resting, usually in concert with increasing disabilities in one or more functional system.
- Levels 6.0 and 6.5 reflect the requirement of unilateral or bilateral assistance for ambulation, respectively.

- Levels 7.0 and 7.5 reflect the need for a wheelchair with or without a requirement for assistance with transfer.
- Levels of 8.0 and above reflect increasingly severe bed- or chair-bound status and increasing dependence on others for all functions.

Major difficulties with the EDSS derive from the fact that while it reflects a continuum of accumulated disability (ordinal data), the steps in the EDSS scale are not necessarily equal (continuous data). This leads to problems in the statistical analysis of group data based on the EDSS. It also leads to some aberrations in the scores assigned to some patients. Finally, because the EDSS has been used to select patients for clinical trials, usually restricting patient's entry based on their ability to walk without assistive devices (level 5.5), or any limitations of endurance (level 5.0), or on their ability to walk at least 5 metres even if bilateral assistance is required (level 6.5), the same criteria have subsequently been artificially imposed by regulatory agencies and third-party payers for limiting the use of newer immunomodulatory drugs to certain MS patient subgroups.

Prognosis at presentation

Often, individuals present with clinical syndromes that are highly suggestive of MS, but a clinically definite diagnosis cannot be established (Table 4.1). These patients include those with monosymptomatic presentations, such as optic neuritis, incomplete spinal-cord syndromes (partial transverse myelitis) and certain brainstem syndromes (internuclear ophthalmoplegia, facial myokymia and isolated limb ataxia). In these individuals, the MRI findings at presentation are useful in assessing the risk of having a disease-defining clinical event and for developing fixed neurological disability over the next 2–5 years. The presence and number of lesions on cerebral MRI is useful in predicting moderate to high risk; the absence of abnormalities on cerebral MRI suggests a low risk of progression to clinically definite disease or modest disability. In the absence of abnormalities on cerebral MRI, the presence or absence of oligoclonal bands in the CSF further refines the risk levels over the next several years. Data are not available to suggest that either MRI or CSF findings are useful prognostic indicators of future disease course for individual patients with clinically definite MS.

CHAPTER 5

Treatment of acute attacks and symptomatic measures

Acute attacks

Corticosteroid therapy is the treatment that has been most convincingly shown to influence either the severity or duration of the acute attack. Controversy remains regarding the most effective type of steroid, and whether the type of steroid used has any influence on the subsequent disease course.

The first properly randomized, double-blind study of steroids for acute exacerbations of MS used adrenocorticotrophic hormone (ACTH) over a 2-week period. The authors concluded that treated patients showed some advantage over non-treated patients in the first 2 weeks, predominantly in terms of motor, sensory and sphincter function. Although the analysis ceased at 4 weeks after entry to the trial, the data suggested that soon afterwards there would have been no significant difference between the two groups. Subsequently, oral steroids were used on the assumption that the oral preparation was as effective as ACTH. Eventually, controlled studies concluded that intravenous methylprednisolone, 500–1000 mg daily for 3–7 days, was superior to placebo, but not necessarily superior to ACTH. Intravenous methylprednisolone hastens return of normal vision in patients with optic neuritis compared with either oral prednisolone or placebo, but without any influence on the long-term outcome in terms of residual visual deficits. More recently, a study of intravenous versus oral methyl-prednisolone failed to demonstrate an advantage of the former over the latter formulation.

A complicating factor when deciding which steroid preparation to use is the evidence that, for some types of attack, the mode of treatment has an influence on the subsequent course of the disease. In one study in which patients with optic neuritis were treated with placebo, oral steroids or intravenous steroids, twice as many patients in the placebo and oral steroid arms developed MS over a 2-year follow-up period compared with the group that received methylprednisolone intravenously at the time of the acute attack. By 4 years' follow up, however, the rate of developing MS was similar in all three treatment groups.

Which patients with acute attacks should be treated? In general, it seems reasonable to confine treatment to those patients whose attacks are disabling, though not necessarily requiring their admission to hospital. If, on the other hand, the attack has not had a significant effect on lifestyle, steroid therapy hardly seems worthwhile.

Symptomatic measures

Fatigue is a common complaint in MS patients. Although studies have suggested that amantadine and possibly pemoline can lessen this symptom, neither drug has been shown to affect attention, visual or verbal memory, or motor speed in a double-blind study of MS patients.

Motor, visual or cerebellar function. Aminopyridines enhance nerve conduction in the central nervous system. 4-aminopyridine has been shown to have some objective effect on extraocular motility, strength, coordination, gait and visual function in MS patients. The effects are small and the drug is not used routinely.

Spasticity. The main drugs used for the treatment of spasticity are baclofen, dantrolene, diazepam and tizanidine (Table 5.1). Baclofen is probably the drug of choice. The starting dose is around 15 mg/day, and this should be increased slowly, otherwise sedation becomes a major problem. Rapid withdrawal of the drug can lead to a rebound increase in spasticity. Diazepam is an alternative agent, but high doses are often required. Clonazepam is sometimes used. Dantrolene acts peripherally. Rarely, striking flaccidity can result with any of these drugs, a disadvantage to the patient if weakness is also a problem. Tizanidine, a drug related to clonidine, has a significant effect on spasticity and is now licensed in the UK as well as the USA.

If oral preparations are unhelpful, and the spasticity is disabling, intrathecal baclofen can be considered. Spasticity is significantly relieved, as are spontaneous spasms and pain. Complications of the technique include wound infection, pump malfunctions and low-pressure headache due to CSF leakage.

Botulinum toxin is, at least theoretically, a potential treatment for spasticity. Objective improvement in spasticity is demonstrable, but

39

TABLE 5.1

Antispasticity agents

	Diazepam	Baclofen
Daily dose	2–15 mg, divided doses	15–100 mg, divided doses
Mode of action	Acts on GABA-mediated inhibitory circuits	Acts as a GABA-agonist at a spinal level
Common side-effects	• Drowsiness • Confusion • Ataxia • Paradoxical increase in aggression • Dependency	• Sedation • Drowsiness • Nausea • Lassitude • Dizziness • Ataxia • Depression • Tremor

considerable quantities of the drug are required for treatment of the leg muscles, and injections are needed every 3 months or so.

The role of physiotherapy, with or without an antispastic agent, has been appraised. There is evidence to suggest that the beneficial effects of baclofen on spasticity can be enhanced by the concomitant use of stretching exercises.

Bladder symptoms are very common in established MS. The most characteristic complaint is of urgency and frequency, sometimes combined with incontinence, but on other occasions with hesitancy and a poor stream. The symptoms are often the result of a mismatch between detrusor contraction and bladder neck relaxation.

Before embarking on drug therapy, an understanding of the type of bladder disorder is essential. Appraisal of symptoms alone is not enough for this purpose and investigation of bladder status is necessary. Ultrasound analysis of the bladder volume pre- and post-micturition is invaluable and may suffice for rational management. In some instances, cystometry is required. The discovery of a large post-micturition residual volume is a relative contraindication to the use of certain drugs (Figure 5.1).

Dantrolene sodium	Tizanidine
25–400 mg, divided doses	2–36 mg, divided doses
Acts peripherally on inhibitory circuits	α_2-adrenoreceptor agonist at a spinal level
• Drowsiness	• Dry mouth
• Dizziness	• Somnolence
• Fatigue	• Asthenia
• Diarrhoea	• Dizziness
• Nausea	• Headache
• Headache	

The currently available drugs act at different sites of the neurogenic pathway that controls micturition (Figure 5.2 and Table 5.2).

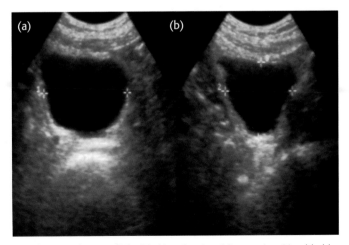

Figure 5.1 Ultrasound scans of the bladder showing (a) pre-micturition bladder and (b) post-micturition bladder with a large post-micturition residual volume. The cursors (+) mark the bladder wall boundaries.

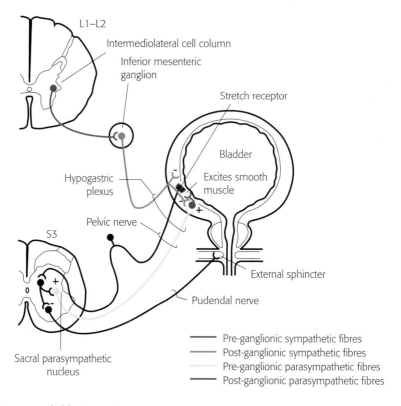

Figure 5.2 Bladder innervation.

Urge incontinence. For patients with urge incontinence (due to detrusor hyperreflexia), the drugs of choice are either oxybutynin (5–15 mg daily, in divided doses), propantheline (30–90 mg daily, in divided doses) or tolterodine (2–4 mg daily, in divided doses). Alternatively, a tricyclic antidepressant (e.g. amitriptyline) may be given as a single dose at night. The use of all these drugs is limited by anticholinergic side-effects (e.g. dry mouth and constipation). If they lead to an increasing urinary residual volume, their use must be reconsidered. Desmopressin, 10–20 μg at night, is helpful in younger patients in whom nocturnal frequency and incontinence is a problem. Care should be taken to avoid fluid overload.

Incomplete emptying. For these patients (e.g. those with residual volume exceeding 100 ml), intermittent catheterization is probably needed. However, before taking this course of action, the patient can try to stimulate bladder

TABLE 5.2

Drugs for bladder symptoms

Drug	Site and mode of action
Anticholinergics (e.g. propantheline, oxybutynin, tolterodine)	Reduce detrusor hyperreflexia
Cholinergics	Enhance detrusor activity
α-sympathetic blockers (e.g. indoramin)	Relax smooth muscle including the internal sphincter
Antispastic agents (e.g. baclofen)	Relax tone in the external sphincter
Vasopressin analogues (e.g. desmopressin)	Reduce urine production (for the management of nocturia)

emptying by stimulating the anal region or the lower abdomen. If this fails, a trial of an α-adrenergic blocking agent (e.g. indoramin, 20–100 mg, daily) is worth considering.

Eventually, intermittent self-catheterization is required if there is a persistent, significant, post-micturition volume. The incidence of bladder infection is far lower than with indwelling or suprapubic catheters. Providing the patient has reasonable vision and hand control, the procedure is readily learned. The patient should be advised to have a high fluid intake.

Urinary tract infections. Despite taking the above measures, urinary tract infections still occur. Urine culture is essential before starting therapy. Many infections respond to either ampicillin, nalidixic acid, nitrofurantoin or trimethoprim, for 1 week. Resistant organisms are common, however. If frequent, symptomatic infections occur, consider long-term, low-dose antibiotic therapy (e.g. trimethoprim or nitrofurantoin, the latter at 50–100 mg at night).

Surgery. When all other measures have failed, various forms of surgical intervention may be used. In one procedure, bladder neck closure is accompanied by the introduction of a suprapubic catheter. Neural prostheses have been used in an attempt to stimulate bladder voiding but have been mainly used in patients with spinal cord trauma.

Bowel problems

Faecal incontinence is relatively uncommon. When present, it usually accompanies urinary urgency and incontinence. Constipation is a more common problem, often compounded by the anticholinergic properties of some of the drugs used for symptom control. Most patients respond to an increase in the fibre in their diet, or to osmotic laxatives, such as lactulose.

Sexual problems

Some of the problems that MS patients experience with sexual intercourse relate either to loss of vaginal or penile sensation, or to the difficulties that spasticity imposes on the physical act itself. Beyond this is the problem of erectile impotence. In the past, the most successful treatment has involved intracavernous injection of vasoactive drugs, such as papaverine. Hazards of the procedure include haematoma formation, local scarring and the induction of prolonged erections. The recently introduced oral agent sildenafil may benefit some patients with erectile impotence.

Depression

Depression is more common in MS patients than is euphoria, and is more common in MS patients than in individuals with other neurological disorders that produce a comparable degree of disability. Its genesis, other than the immediate conclusion that it is triggered by a reaction to the illness itself, remains unknown. The evidence that bipolar depression is more common in the MS population is not persuasive. Management is the same as it is for depression occurring under other circumstances, though larger doses of tricyclic antidepressants may well produce troublesome side-effects.

Some patients exhibit pathological laughter and crying, which may respond to lower doses of amitriptyline.

Tremor

A severe, upper limb tremor, particularly of the dominant hand, can lead to substantial disability. Drug therapy, for example with propranolol, is of only limited value. The roles of thalamotomy and thalamic pacing

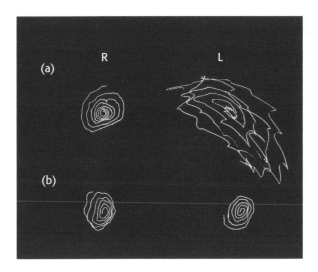

Figure 5.3 Spiral drawn by an MS patient with tremor (a) before and (b) after right thalamotomy.

with implanted electrodes are being resurrected in the management of this problem. Stereotactic lesions in the thalamus can have a dramatic effect on tremor without contributing to the other disabilities of the limb (Figure 5.3).

Pain

Various types of pain occur in MS patients, other than trigeminal neuralgia. A chronic aching discomfort of the lower limbs occurs in patients with myelopathy and may respond to amitriptyline. Sometimes burning dysaesthesiae occur, either in the lower limbs or in the perineal region. Management of these pain problems is notoriously difficult and best achieved through the multidisciplinary approach of a pain clinic.

CHAPTER 6
Treatment with immunomodulators

Until recently, there were no approved drugs to reduce the frequency of future MS attacks or the probability of accumulating neurological disability over time. Two classes of immunomodulatory drugs are now available:
- type I interferons (IFNs)
- glatiramer acetate (co-polymer-1).

Both drug classes reduce the risk of future attacks, and both may also slow the rate of acquisition of neurological deficits. A third class of immuno-therapy, intravenously administered pooled human immunoglobulin G (IVIG), may have a similar benefit.

Interferons

Interferons are produced naturally by the body. They were first recognized for their role in limiting certain viral infections. Interferons also alter the expression of surface molecules on, and the range of substances secreted by, immune cells. Many of these immunobiological effects of IFNs, while not antigen specific, are potentially relevant to MS. A number of placebo-controlled clinical trials have been performed with different recombinant IFN molecules. In general, the type I IFNs (IFNα and IFNβ) reduce clinical relapse frequency, while type II IFNs (IFNγ) provoke attacks in MS. The larger, published, pivotal trials were limited to several forms of recombinant IFNβ. All of these were conducted in ambulatory patients with remitting relapsing disease and varying amounts of clinical disability. Several trials are just concluding on ambulatory patients with secondary progressive MS.

Trials. Trial designs differed between the pivotal trials (Table 6.1). Individual studies randomized between 301 and 560 patients, who were then followed with varying success for 18 months to up to 5 years, in controlled fashion. Study end-points differed from a primary emphasis on attack rates to a focus on progression of sustained disability. MRI monitoring differed in frequency and whether the presence of gadolinium-enhanced lesions was available for use as a supportive outcome variable. Comparisons between trials are difficult at best, and the original publications for each trial should be read carefully. The major clinical outcomes of these studies are summarized in Table 6.1. All studies found at least some, and in some cases considerable, evidence to support the clinical benefits observed by analysis of MRI measures of lesion burden and disease activity. Smaller studies using frequent gadolinium-enhanced MRI for monitoring show that institution of treatment with IFN at appropriate doses rapidly reduces enhanced lesion frequency. This MRI-monitored effect is lost when IFN treatment is withdrawn.

A trial of rIFNβ-1b in secondary progressive MS that used the time to sustained progression of disability as its primary study outcome was recently stopped. Early termination of the trial was based on a planned interim analysis that reportedly favoured active treatment. A similar trial of rIFNβ-1a has been completed with less impressive effects on progression. Other trials are still ongoing. The results of these important studies should better define the range of severity of MS that may benefit from immunotherapy with IFNs.

Side-effect profiles of the three IFNβ preparations vary according to dose and route of administration. All of the preparations are associated with flu-like side-effects, including fever, malaise, joint and muscle pain, and these appear to be dose dependent. The first injections may result in a transient worsening of neurological function that is probably related to the Uhthoff effect (transient deterioration of current or reappearance of prior neurological deficits in association with elevated body temperature). The intensity of these reactions usually attenuates rapidly with subsequent injections. Reactions at the injection site are common when IFNs are administered subcutaneously. They range from local redness at the injection site with or without itching, to local induration of variable duration and severity, to local skin necrosis (Figure 6.1). The last is uncommon, and is sometimes the consequence of unintended intracutaneous injections. Skin reactions and injection-associated flu-like symptoms usually decrease over time, but remain major causes of early patient non-compliance. Lymphopenia and hepatic enzyme elevations are also dose-dependent side-effects of therapy. These seldom necessitate discontinuation of IFN treatment. Less common later effects of therapy are exacerbation or unmasking of psoriasis and development of hypothyroidism.

TABLE 6.1

Results of pivotal trials in remitting relapsing MS

Type	References	Proprietary name	Weekly dose*
Type I interferons			
IFNβ-1b	IFNB MS Study Group 1993	Betaseron®/ Betaferon®	0
			175 µg subcutaneously
			875 µg subcutaneously
IFNβ-1a	Jacobs *et al.* 1996	Avonex®	0
			33 µg intramuscularly
	PRISMS Study Group 1998	Rebif®	0
			66 µg subcutaneously
			132 µg subcutaneously
Glatiramer acetate			
	Johnson *et al.* 1995	Copaxone®	0
			140 mg subcutaneously
Pooled human immunoglobulin G			
	Fazekas *et al.* 1997	IVIG	0
			0.2 g/kg/month

*Weekly dose in mass; note: the biological activities of IFNβ-1b and IFNβ-1a cannot be compared directly on a mass basis, the bioavailability of an equivalent mass of the two IFNβ-1a may differ according to route of administration

†Annual relapse rate based on an intention-to-treat analysis of the data

‡Patients improved or worsened by ≥ 1.0 on the extended disability status score (EDSS) at the conclusion of the trial compared with their entry EDSS level

Glatiramer acetate

Glatiramer (co-polymer-1; Copaxone®) binds strongly to molecules on the surfaces of antigen-presenting cells, which are central to the induction of antigen-specific immune responses. In animals, the drug may prevent immune-mediated neurological disease through the induction of organ-specific immunoregulatory T cells. Similar mechanisms may account for its effects in MS.

Relapse rate[†]	Improved (%)[‡]	Worsened (%)[‡]	Progressed (%)[§]	NtAb (%)[¶]
1.27	NA	39	28	–
1.17	NA	35	28	42
0.84	NA	27	20	38
0.82	12	36	35	–
0.67	19	24	22	14
1.33	13	32	39	–
0.94	19	25	30	26
0.92	16	26	27	17
0.81	12	31	42	–
0.58	27	18	22	–
1.26	14	23	NA	–
0.52	31	17	NA	–

[§]Patients who progressed: for IFNs, ≥ 1.0 units from their baseline EDSS and sustained this deterioration for 3–6 months; for glatiramer acetate, ≥ 1.5 units from baseline EDSS exclusive of relapses

[¶]Patients who developed IFN neutralizing antibodies that may be at risk for loss of benefit from continued treatment

NtAB = neutralizing antibodies; NA = not available from data presented in the publications

Trials. Several small, controlled studies suggested that glatiramer reduced the frequency of attacks and decreased accumulation of neurological disease, particularly in remitting relapsing MS patients with limited neurological disability. A large multicentre study that was extended in controlled fashion for an average of 33 months confirmed these findings (see Table 6.1). The observed annualized attack rates, proportion of attack-free subjects, number of subjects improved over the course of the trial and proportion of patients

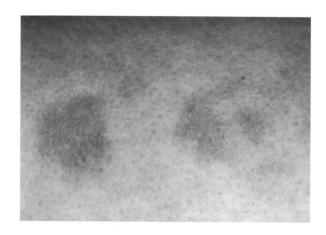

Figure 6.1
Skin reaction to subcutaneous injection of interferon.

progressing without acute attacks were reduced by active drug therapy. The effects of glatiramer on MRI-monitored disease parameters parallel the clinical results.

Side-effects. Few side-effects are seen with glatiramer therapy. Transient pain and/or minor swelling at the injection sites are common at the onset of therapy, but these rapidly attenuate with time (Figure 6.2). Skin necrosis is not encountered. Neither flu-like side-effects nor laboratory abnormalities occur. However, 10–15% of patients treated with glatiramer will eventually experience one or more 'systemic post-injection reactions'. During these reactions, patients report varied combinations of flushing, sweating, palpitations, a feeling of chest tightness and associated anxiety. The

Figure 6.2
Reaction to glatiramer therapy at injection site.

symptom complex usually resolves in a few minutes but rarely lasts several hours. These reactions are temporally associated with injection of the drug, are not seen with the first injection and do not occur on successive injections. They appear to be benign, but the mechanism of induction of the systemic post-injection reaction remains uncertain. Preclinical studies in animals suggest that glatiramer is neither toxic nor teratogenic.

Intravenous immunoglobulin

Several small, controlled trials suggest that pooled human immunoglobulin given monthly by intravenous infusion may decrease relapse frequency and reduce accumulated disability in patients with remitting relapsing MS. Early results of MRI-monitoring of this treatment suggest a modest effect on gadolinium-enhancement frequency. Cost, convenience, side-effects and the potential to transmit adventitious agents may limit the general use of this form of therapy to selected patients who fail to respond to IFN or glatiramer.

Summary

Considerable evidence, most from controlled clinical trials, supports the use of rIFNβ for the treatment of relapsing forms of MS. For those patients who tolerate this form of therapy and who do not develop sustained high titres of neutralizing antibody, a reduction in clinical relapses and MRI-monitored disease activity can be expected, and a slowing of accumulated clinical and MRI-measured disease burden anticipated. The best protection appears to be afforded by the higher dose formulations, but even lower dose preparations have effects on these disease parameters.

The use of glatiramer acetate is supported by several independent studies and the effect of the drug on MRI-measured disease parameters was recently established. Reduction in the number of clinical attacks and slowing of clinical disability is anticipated when the drug is used in ambulatory, relapsing patients with mild-to-moderate clinical disability.

Monthly infusions of immunoglobulin also appear to reduce the frequency of attacks in those patients with remitting relapsing disease, and may slow the accumulation of neurological disability. This therapy is not amenable to self-administration. The use of any drug class in patients with secondary progressive disease is not as well defined, but higher doses of IFN probably modestly slow progressive accumulation of disabilities. The benefits of immunotherapy in patients with primary progressive disease is untested. Nevertheless, the data increasingly support the early use of either IFNβ or glatiramer acetate in patients with clinically definite relapsing MS.

CHAPTER 7

Paramedical staff and support groups

Doctors have become increasingly aware of the need to understand their patient's perception of their own lifestyle and what measures, through the intervention of paramedical staff, might be taken to enhance its quality. A number of studies of quality of life among MS patients have been performed. Though conclusions are difficult to draw from these appraisals (differing test formats have been applied), the patients have generally scored poorly in certain areas – particularly physical functioning and energy/ vitality – both in comparison with patients with other chronic diseases and in comparison with healthy controls.

Attempts to modify the patient's level of disability can be considered either through the aegis of in-patient rehabilitation, or through concerted action by various paramedical staff on an out-patient basis.

In-patient rehabilitation

In-patient rehabilitation, by definition, will be multidisciplinary. Healthcare professionals will aim to devise a programme of therapy that fits the patient's needs and is thoroughly understood and approved by the patient. The exact value of such rehabilitation remains uncertain, not least because of the various outcome measures proposed to measure the benefit of any intervention, and because of the multifactorial nature of the influences that might affect outcome.

Studies have suggested that MS patients benefit from in-patient rehabilitation in various aspects of everyday life, including self-care activities, transfers and homemaking skills. These benefits, it is suggested, are not simply confined to those patients showing a reduction in neurological impairment during the rehabilitation period. Analysis of the ongoing nature of any benefit achieved during the in-patient rehabilitation period suggests it may well depend on the therapeutic input achieved following discharge.

Community care

In both the UK and USA, the prevalence of MS approximates to 100 per 100 000, one-half of whom are estimated to be disabled. Disability, in this context, refers to any restriction or lack of ability to perform any activity of everyday living. Handicap is defined as a disadvantage, arising out of a particular disability, that limits or prevents an individual from performing a particular role in society. Though the individual contributions of the paramedical team are now discussed, their integration as a seamless service is of vital importance to the patient's welfare.

Physiotherapist. In addition to drug therapy for the management of spasticity, the intervention of a physiotherapist is of value in its assessment and treatment. Spasticity is enhanced by noxious stimuli from bladder infection, pressure sores or faecal impaction. Management of these problems alone can considerably reduce the level of spasticity or flexor spasms. Stretch exercises on spastic muscles diminish spasticity for some hours after the therapy and, if performed regularly, will inhibit the development of flexor spasms. Management of ataxia is difficult. Measures can be taken to compensate for ataxia using visual and sensory guidance though in many MS sufferers, multifocal disability inhibits the use of such compensatory mechanisms. Regular input from the physiotherapist is valuable for refreshing techniques for the activities of daily living.

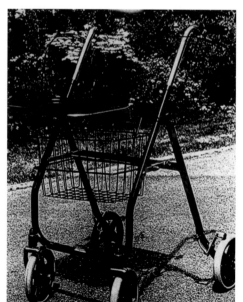

Figure 7.1 A walking frame can be used as walking ability declines. The Rambler Walking Frame is shown with permission from Boots, UK.

TABLE 7.1

The modified Barthel activities of daily living index

Bowels

0   Incontinent or needs enemata

1   Occasional accident

2   Continent

Bladder

0   Incontinent or catheterized

1   Occasional accident

2   Continent for > 7 days

Grooming

0   Needs help with personal care

1   Independent with aids if necessary

Toilet use

0   Dependent

1   Needs some help

2   Fully independent

Feeding

0   Unable

1   Needs help

2   Independent

Transfers

0   Unable, no sitting balance

1   Major help (one or two people, physical); can sit

2   Minor help (verbal or physical)

3   Independent

Mobility

0   Immobile

1   Wheelchair-independent

2   Walks with help of one person

3   Independent with aids if necessary

Dressing

0   Dependent

1   Needs help

2   Independent

Stairs

0   Unable

1   Needs help

2   Independent

Bathing

0   Dependent

1   Independent

Total

0–4 = very severely disabled

5–9 = severely disabled

10–14 = moderately disabled

15–19 = mildly disabled

20 = physically independent, but not necessarily normal or socially independent

Occupational therapist. The occupational therapist is particularly involved in assessments of daily living (ADL) with a view to determining areas of difficulty, and then seeking, by the use of modified techniques or aids, to improve function in that area and promote independence. The Barthel index is widely used in this context (Table 7.1). The index does not cover certain critical activities, for example cooking and communication, so additional test systems may be needed to obtain a full picture of the patient's disability.

Areas in which appliances may prove of value include adapted cutlery and dressing and bathing aids. For more severely disabled patients, environment control systems can maintain independence. As walking deteriorates, various walking appliances can be introduced (Figure 7.1), culminating eventually in the use of a wheelchair. Choice of chair is critical and will be influenced by whether the chair is for indoor or outdoor use, what additional appliances need to be attached to the chair, and whether the chair is propelled by the patient, a carer or electronically (Figure 7.2). Many disabled patients can continue to drive, providing that they use an appropriately adapted car and have received instruction at a specialized assessment centre (see page 62).

Speech and swallow therapists. Both dysarthria and dysphagia occur in patients with MS. Speech therapy may enable the patient to find various strategies to help compensate for a cerebellar dysarthria. Communication aids are only likely to help those patients with reasonably intact vision and upper limb coordination (Figure 7.3).

Swallow function is best assessed by carrying out a timed analysis of swallowing fluids and boluses of differing consistency abetted by videofluoroscopy. Sucking ice prior to eating may lessen bulbar spasticity while altering posture during swallowing can reduce laryngeal penetration.

Social worker. The social worker can often provide, with the physician, a focus for the patient's ongoing care. In addition to this, he or she is well placed to assess the effect of the patient's illness both on the patient and the family unit. They are able to advise on financial matters, and can integrate any hospital care with the appropriate community services. Together with the occupational therapist, he or she can advise on housing needs. Together with the family physician, a social worker can develop a care-package

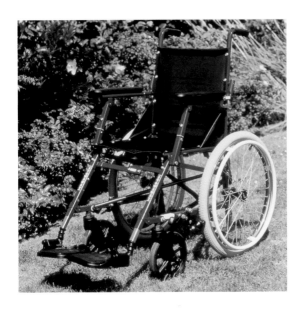

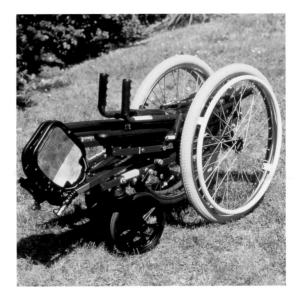

Figure 7.2 A wheelchair that collapses when not in use can be particularly convenient for patients who travel regularly. Reproduced with permission from Smith and Nephew Homecraft Limited, UK.

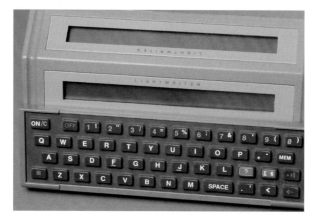

Figure 7.3 A communication aid. Reproduced with permission from Easi Aids, UK.

programme for the more disabled patient. This will integrate various components of a home-support system and provide advice on the benefits of attendance at day centres that cater for MS patients or the value of periodic in-patient stays linked with an active rehabilitation programme.

Psychologist. Although it is often assumed that cognitive difficulties occur only in the later stages of MS, and then correlate with measures of physical disability, neither premise is correct. There is little correlation between cognitive impairment and disease duration, or with other measures of neurological impairment. Cognitive impairment is a predictor of handicap, and an indicator that the patient will eventually become dependent. Problems with abstract reasoning, memory and attention will interfere with the patient's understanding of their condition and their capacity to make decisions for the future. The potential to benefit from rehabilitation programmes is likely to be correspondingly diminished.

Specialist nurse. The concept of a specialist nurse with a particular interest and expertise for one aspect of neurological disability has led to them working in fields such as MS, epilepsy and Parkinson's disease. A specialist nurse can provide input following initial diagnosis, discuss aspects of care (including the use of new drugs) with the patient and liaise with the family physician and the hospital service as new needs are identified.

The MS Society provides, for patients in the UK, a valuable resource of information and guidance (see Appendix). Objective advice on the many issues relating to the disease are available, for example in relation to diet, the role of IFNβ and discussion on the various symptoms encountered by patients. Patients can receive advice on benefits and on local networks of the society, which can then provide support on a 'one-to-one' basis. In the USA, a similar function is provided by the National Multiple Sclerosis Society (NMSS) and its many chapters.

The Disabled Living Foundation serves as a source of information for patients with disabilities, and for those professional staff dealing with them (see Appendix). The foundation has a reference library and a comprehensive information service. Over 30 Disabled Living Centres have been established in the UK, where aids can be assessed by the patient, backed, in most instances, by expert advice. In addition, the centres hold meetings and study days to broaden knowledge among care workers and concerned individuals dealing with people with MS or other conditions associated with ongoing disability.

CHAPTER 8

Future trends

Advances in both basic and applied research into MS over the past few decades have been substantial, and the application of new investigative techniques promises to further shape our understanding of this for long enigmatic disease.

Aetiology

Available data confirm there is an immunopathogenic component to the disease process of MS. Whether the immune mechanisms are primary in the pathogenesis or reflect a response to a persistent CNS infection in which nervous system tissue is damaged secondarily by an otherwise well-directed immune response is difficult to determine. The continued application of modern molecular techniques should establish the importance of any persistent CNS infection in directing a secondary immunopathogenic response. It is also likely that as more specific and effective immuno-modulatory therapies are developed, explaining incomplete responses to immunomodulatory therapies by an ongoing, persistent CNS infection will be rendered *passé*.

Several independent studies to identify the genetic profiles that confer disease susceptibility in members of multiplex MS families have been relatively disappointing. It is likely, however, that a considerable proportion of the clinical phenotypic variation common in MS will be explained by the genotype profiles which control patterns of immune expression at the cellular level, such as the proportions and amounts of chemokines and cytokines secreted on immune activation. Thus, monophasic demyelinating diseases, relapsing forms of MS associated with little acquired disability over decades, rapidly progressive forms of the disease, and perhaps primary progressive phenotypes may be better characterized early on by determination of such genetic profiles.

Diagnosis and disease staging

MRI has contributed substantially to our understanding of the dynamics of the disease process, and has also proved useful in diagnosis. Extensive experience with MRI means that current diagnostic criteria, based on the suggestions of the Washington panel, require updating. Certain patterns on cerebral and spinal MRI may allow MS to be diagnosed in the absence of classical recurrent clinical attacks, and possibly in the absence of clinical symptoms. New diagnostic criteria for primary progressive MS will undoubtedly incorporate MRI findings. However, better information is still needed to understand patients with clinically definite and laboratory-supported MS in whom neuro-imaging of the entire neural axis is normal.

Therapy

As more sophisticated imaging approaches are introduced into clinical practice, including the more routine use of magnetic resonance spectroscopic imaging, imaging profiles specific to biologically meaningful clinical disease phenotypes and genotypes, with both prognostic and therapeutic implications, are likely to emerge. An increasing number of signatures of the effects of different drugs on MRI, such as a profound effect of IFNs on enhancement that exceeds their clinical benefit or the delayed effects of glatiramer acetate on enhancement that mirror its clinical effects, are also likely to be seen. Differences in both the apparent mechanisms of action and MRI signatures of various new immunomodulatory agents may allow for the rational choice of drugs for individual patients, and for the informed study of combined therapies. It is also possible that recent reports of antibody-stimulated remyelination will lead to the discovery of effective small-peptide ligands that stimulate oligodendroglial cell regeneration, ushering in therapeutic trials with an end-point of clinical improvement, rather than slowing disease progression.

Key references

EPIDEMIOLOGY, PATHOLOGY AND PATHOPHYSIOLOGY

Lindsey JW, Wolinsky JS. Demyelinating diseases. In: Dale DC, Federman DD, eds. *Scientific American Medicine*. New York: Scientific American Medicine Inc., 1997:1–11.

Paty DW, Ebers GC, eds. *Multiple Sclerosis*. Philadelphia: FA Davis Company, 1998.

Raine CS, McFarland HF, Tourtellotte WW, eds. *Multiple Sclerosis: Clinical and Pathogenetic Basis*. London: Chapman & Hall, 1997.

Rudick RA, Cohen JA, Weinstock-Guttman B *et al*. Management of multiple sclerosis. *N Engl J Med* 1997;337: 1604–11.

Sadovnick AD, Baird PA, Ward RH. Multiple sclerosis: updated risks for relatives. *Am J Med Genet* 1988;29: 533–41.

Trapp BD, Peterson J, Ransohoff RM *et al*. Axonal transection in the lesions of multiple sclerosis. *N Engl J Med* 1998; 338:278–85.

CLASSIFICATION, PRESENTATION AND EARLY STAGES

Lublin FD, Reingold SC. Defining the clinical course of multiple sclerosis: results of an international survey. *Neurology* 1996;46:907–11.

Twomey JA, Espir MLE. Paroxysmal symptoms as the first manifestation of multiple sclerosis. *J Neurol Neurosurg Psychiatry* 1980;43:269–304.

Weinshenker BG, Bass B, Rice GPA *et al*. The natural history of multiple sclerosis: a geographically based study: 1. Clinical course and disability. *Brain* 1989;112: 133–46.

THE ESTABLISHED CONDITION

Runmarker B, Andersen O. Prognostic factors in a multiple sclerosis incidence cohort with twenty-five years of follow-up. *Brain* 1993;116:117–34.

Vickrey BG, Hays RD, Harouni R *et al*. A health-related quality of life measure for multiple sclerosis. *Qual Life Res* 1995;4:187–206.

DIAGNOSIS

Filippi M, Horsfield MA, Ader HJ *et al*. Guidelines for using quantitative measures of brain magnetic resonance imaging abnormalities in monitoring the treatment of multiple sclerosis. *Ann Neurol* 1998;43:499–506.

Filippi M, Yousry T, Baratti C *et al*. Quantitative assessment of MRI lesion load in multiple sclerosis – a comparison of conventional spin-echo with fast fluid-attenuated inversion recovery. *Brain* 1996;119:1349–55.

Kurtzke JF. Rating neurologic impairment in multiple sclerosis: an expanded disability status scale (EDSS). *Neurology* 1983;33:1444–52.

Poser CM, Paty DW, Scheinberg L *et al*. New diagnostic criteria for multiple sclerosis: guidelines for research protocols. *Ann Neurol* 1983;13:227–31.

Schumacher GA, Beebe G, Kibler RF *et al.* Problems of experimental trials of therapy in multiple sclerosis: report by the panel on the evaluation of experimental trials of therapy in multiple sclerosis. *Ann NY Acad Sci* 1965;122:522–69.

Soederstroem M, Ya-Ping J, Hillert J *et al.* Optic neuritis – prognosis for multiple sclerosis from MRI, CSF and HLA findings. *Neurology* 1998;50:708–14.

Van Walderveen MAA, Barkhof F, Hommes OR *et al.* Correlating MRI and clinical disease activity in multiple sclerosis: relevance of hypointense lesions on short-TR/short-TE (T1-weighted) spin-echo images. *Neurology* 1995;45:1684–90.

Whitaker JN, McFarland HF, Rudge P *et al.* Outcomes assessment in multiple sclerosis clinical trials: a critical analysis. *MS Clin Lab Res* 1995;1:37–47.

TREATMENT OF ACUTE ATTACKS AND SYMPTOMATIC MEASURES

Barnes D, Hughes RAC, Morris RW *et al.* Randomised trial of oral and intravenous methyl prednisolone in acute relapses of multiple sclerosis. *Lancet* 1997;349:902–6.

Fowler CJ, Van Kerrebroeck PE, Nordeno A *et al.* Treatment of lower urinary tract dysfunction in patients with multiple sclerosis. Committee of the European Study Group of SUDIMS (Sexual and Urological Disorders in Multiple Sclerosis). *J Neurol Neurosurg Psychiatry* 1992;55:986–9.

TREATMENT WITH IMMUNOMODULATORS

Duquette P, Girard M, Dubois R *et al.* Neutralizing antibodies during the treatment of multiple sclerosis with interferon beta-1b: experience during the first three years. *Neurology* 1996;47:889–94.

Ebers GC, Rice G, Lesaux J *et al.* Randomised double-blind placebo-controlled study of interferon beta-1a in relapsing/remitting multiple sclerosis. PRISMS (Prevention of Relapses and Disability by Interferon beta-1a Subcutaneously in Multiple Sclerosis) Study Group. *Lancet* 1998;352:1498–504.

Fazekas F, Deisenhammer F, Strasser-Fuchs S *et al.* Randomised placebo-controlled trial of monthly intravenous immunoglobulin therapy in relapsing-remitting multiple sclerosis. *Lancet* 1997;349:589–93.

IFNB Multiple Sclerosis Study Group. Interferon beta-1b is effective in relapsing-remitting multiple sclerosis. I. Clinical results of a multicenter, randomized, double-blind, placebo-controlled trial. *Neurology* 1993;43:655–61.

IFNB Multiple Sclerosis Study Group, Univ Brit Columbia MS MRI Analysis Group. Interferon beta-1b in the treatment of multiple sclerosis: final outcome of the randomized controlled trial. *Neurology* 1995;45:1277–85.

Jacobs L, Cookfair DL, Rudick RA *et al.* Intramuscular interferon beta-1a for disease progression in relapsing multiple sclerosis. *Ann Neurol* 1996;39:285–94.

Johnson KP, Brooks BR, Cohen JA *et al.* Copolymer 1 reduces relapse rate and improves disability in relapsing-remitting multiple sclerosis: results of a phase III multicenter, double-blind, placebo-controlled trial. *Neurology* 1995;45: 1268–76.

Johnson KP, Brooks BR, Cohen JA *et al.* Extended use of glatiramer acetate (Copaxone) is well tolerated and maintains its clinical effect on multiple sclerosis relapse rate and degree of disability. *Neurology* 1998;50:701–8.

PARAMEDICAL STAFF AND SUPPORT GROUPS

Fuller KJ, Dawson K, Wiles CM. Physiotherapy in chronic multiple sclerosis: a controlled trial. *Clin Rehabil* 1996;10:195–204.

Kirker SGB, Young E, Warlow CP. An evaluation of a multiple sclerosis liaison nurse. *Clin Rehabil* 1995;9:219–26.

Index

ACTH 38
acute attacks 38–9
adhesion molecules 10
adrenocorticotrophic
  hormone see ACTH
age and MS 7, 8, 18, 19,
  20, 23
amantadine 39
aminopyridine 39
anaesthetics and MS 29
astrocytes 8, 9, 13
ataxia 21, 24, 27, 28, 37,
  40, 54

B cells 13
baclofen 39, 40
bladder symptoms see
  micturition, altered
blood–brain barrier 8, 10, 12
bowel disturbance 19, 36, 44
brain
  demyelinated plaques 7, 8
  sclerotic lesions 7

carbamazepine 20
central nervous system
  see CNS
cerebellar function 28, 36,
  39, 56
cerebrospinal fluid see CSF
chemokines 10
classifying MS 14–24
clonazepam 39
CNS 9, 31, 32
  inflammatory foci 7
  plaques 8, 13
cognition 8, 27, 58
  see also mental function
community care 53–9
computed tomography see CT
coordination 15
corticosteroids 20, 38
CSF 12, 18, 31, 34–5, 37
CT 21, 22
cytokines 10, 13

daily living index 55, 56
dantrolene 39, 41
demyelination 7, 8–9, 9–13,
  19, 31
depression 21, 27, 40, 44
diagnosis 5, 31–7, 60–1
  clinical criteria 31, 32
    Schumacher 31
    Washington Panel 31, 32
  laboratory criteria 34–5
  paraclinical criteria 31–4
diazepam 39, 40
diet and MS 29–30
Disabled Living Foundation
  (UK) 59, 62
DR molecules 7, 9
driving and MS 30

early stages 5, 14–24
EDSS 35–7, 48, 49
electrophysiological testing
  31–2
epidemiology 7–8
erectile impotence 28, 29, 44
established MS 25–30
expanded disability status
  score see EDSS

fatigue 14, 34, 39, 41
future trends 60–1
  aetiology 60
  diagnosis and staging 60–1
  therapy 61

gender and MS 7, 8, 23
genetic background and MS
  7–8, 29, 60
geography and MS 7
glatiramer acetate 5, 48–52,
  61
  side-effects 50–1
gliosis 8, 9, 13

IFNs 5, 12, 46–8, 51–2, 61
  side-effects 47, 50

immune system 9
immune-mediated component
  7
immunochemical abnormality
  34–5
immunoglobulin G 35, 48, 51
immunological abnormality
  34–5
immunomodulatory drugs 36,
  46–52, 61
intellectual function
  see mental function
interferon drugs see IFNs

macrophages 8–9, 12
magnetic resonance imaging
  see MRI
mental function 36
  altered 21, 26–7, 36
methylprednisolone 38
micturition, altered 16, 19,
  23, 27, 29, 36, 44
  drug therapy 40–3
  surgery 43
motor function 8, 15, 27, 28,
  32, 38, 39
MRI 5, 12, 14, 17, 20, 21, 31,
  32–4, 37, 46–7, 51, 61
MS Society (UK) 59, 62, 63
myelin 8, 13, 35
  antigens 9, 10

National MS Society (USA) 59
neuro-imaging see MRI
neurophysiological testing 31,
  32

oligodendrocytes 9
oligodendroglial cells 8, 9,
  12–13, 61
optic nerve involvement 18,
  19, 33
  demyelinated plaques 7, 8
optic neuritis 17, 24, 27, 32,
  37, 38

pain 17, 18, 20, 21, 30, 45, 47, 50
paraesthesiae 16, 18, 21
paramedical staff 53–9
pathology 8–9
pathophysiology 9–13, 14
pemoline 39
plaques 7, 8, 13, 33, 34
prednisolone 12, 38
pregnancy and MS 29
primary progressive disease 14, 19, 23–4, 25, 52
prodromal symptoms 14
prognosis 37
progressive relapsing disease 14, 24

rehabilitation 53, 58
relapse 22, 26, 32, 49
  see also progressive relapsing disease; remitting relapsing disease
remitting relapsing disease 14–21, 25, 34, 46, 48, 49–50, 51
  definition 14–16
  progression 21
  symptoms 15–21
    paroxysmal 20, 21
remyelination 9, 13, 61

secondary progressive disease 14, 21–3, 26, 46, 51
sensory perception 8, 32, 34, 36, 38
side-effects of therapy 39, 40
  see also glatiramer acetate; IFNs
sodium channels 9
spasticity 20, 27, 28, 39–40, 44, 54, 56
sphincter function 19, 29, 38
spinal cord 18, 32, 33
  demyelinated plaques 7, 8
  dysfunction 23, 37
staging 35–7, 60–1
staining techniques 10–11, 12
steroids see ACTH; corticosteroids; and others by name

support groups 59, 62–3
symptomatic measures 39–45

T cells 8, 9–10, 13, 48
tizanidine 39, 41
trauma and MS 29
tremor 40, 44–5

useful addresses 62–3

vaccinations and MS 29
vertigo 16, 19
viral infections 9, 13
visual involvement 15, 16, 17, 18, 19, 20, 27–8, 30, 36, 37, 39

weakness 16–17, 20, 23
white matter 7, 8, 12, 13, 32, 33, 34

Other titles available in the *Fast Facts* series

Asthma
by Stephen T Holgate and Romain A Pauwels

Allergic Rhinitis
by Niels Mygind and Glenis K Scadding

Benign Prostatic Hyperplasia (third edition)
by Roger S Kirby and John D McConnell

Coeliac Disease
by Geoffrey Holmes and Carlo Catassi

Contraception
by Anna Glasier and Beverly Winikoff

Diseases of the Testis
by Timothy J Christmas, Michael D Dinneen and Larry Lipshultz

Dyspepsia
by Michael J Lancaster Smith and Kenneth L Koch

Endometriosis
by Hossam Abdalla and Botros Rizk

Epilepsy
by Martin J Brodie and Steven C Schachter

Headaches
by Richard Peatfield and J Keith Campbell

Hyperlipidaemia
by Paul Durrington and Allan Sniderman

Irritable Bowel Syndrome
by Kenneth W Heaton and W Grant Thompson

Menopause
by David H Barlow and Barry G Wren

Stress and Strain
by Cary L Cooper and James Campbell Quick

Urinary Continence
by Julian Shah and Gary Leach

To order, please contact:

Health Press Limited
Elizabeth House, Queen Street,
Abingdon, Oxford OX14 3JR, UK
Tel: +44 (0)1235 523233
Fax: +44 (0)1235 523238
Email: post@healthpress.co.uk

Or visit our website:
www.healthpress.co.uk

Health Press
medical publishing at its best

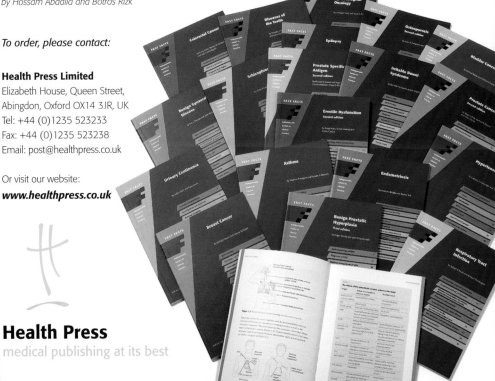